THIS NOTEBOOK BELONGS TO

MISTER & MISSY

Cox

029 005513

adamchoke@gmail

5/2017 – 01/2020

credit karma
mission credit confidence

credence RM

Made in the USA
Middletown, DE
01 April 2022

63475030R00070